Quitting Social Media

The Social Media Cleanse Guide

Lidiya K

How to Stop Using Social Media Copyright © 2018

ISBN: 9781977036704

Warning and Disclaimer

Publisher Contact

Skinny Bottle Publishing

books@skinnybottle.com

Introduction

I like exploring successful people's lives. It's exciting to see how they started from nothing and got to the top, the life lessons they learned, the mistakes they made which we can avoid, and the many obstacles they overcame.

But the real formula for their achievements lies in how they spend their days. What the most productive individuals and famous entrepreneurs do first thing in the morning, how they get ready to get to work, what they do in their free time, how they communicate, what tools they use, how they structure their day, and - ultimately - how they end it. All this is what we should learn from if we want to see a change in our life too.

After getting familiar with the daily routines of many of them over the years, I started noticing some tendencies.

They all had morning and evening routines that helped them stay on track. Each, of course, was a result of years of experimentation until they found the right combination of habits and activities to help them be their best, every day.

There's also the ability to be laser-focused when you're working, but to completely empty your mind when you're not. And with a little research, it turns out longer hours don't necessarily lead to increased productivity.

What's going on in their mind when they look at their to-do list and decide to get done the very first item on top, instead of feeling overwhelmed about the big picture, is an example of discipline and great personal organization.

There's a reason I'm sharing all this. And that's what all the actions and thoughts of successful people have in common, and what prevents the average ones from ever improving their life.

It's all about attention.

Even if you've tried to take control over different aspects of your life, chances are you still rely on plenty of outer factors. That's true for your relationships, career, the place you live, the vacations you take, the things you do when you're free, and so on.

But the one thing you do control, and which might be your biggest asset, is attention.

What you pay attention to at any moment is key to where you end up in life some time from now.

Let me give you some examples.

We often assume we decide how we spend our time, but if we analyze the last few days, and what we were doing in our free time, we'll see it's not like that. Maybe you decided to just relax, but then someone messages you, you receive an email and must act upon it, or just overthink what happened at work.

Or maybe you are trying to hack the whole time management thing, but still, the biggest problem is getting in the zone when working. And due to the many, many distractions in your mind and around you, that takes you longer than it's supposed to. So, you're still wasting a ton of time weekly just trying to get concentrated before work, and again after each break you take.

There are dozens of situations like that daily. The result is that countless factors are fighting for our attention. If we're just living life unconsciously, we give in to each temptation and do things we don't really want or should do, but which are just brought to our attention in the present moment and we don't question that.

However, in the long-run, a life lived like that is filled with regrets.

Even if you set goals such as starting a business on the side, going the extra mile at work to finally get that promotion, breaking an unhealthy habit, taking up a new sport, finally following your passion, learning a new skill, or else, you won't succeed in it without having full control over your attention.

And that's why I'm writing this book.

I want you to get your attention back and invest it in better things, that will truly give you satisfaction and make you feel good about yourself and what you're doing at the end of the day.

The purpose of this series is to help you have a new beginning. As you may know, new beginnings are the hardest. It takes some time and quite a lot of willpower and focus to get there, but it's worth it as then you'll be living life on your own terms.

One of the most interesting things about beginnings is this. You turn over a new leaf in one area of your life, and suddenly, everything else is improved too. During the process, you build some personal qualities, habits and mental patterns that will later come in handy with any endeavor you set your mind to.

Change is great. Those who stay away from it, live without any excitement. They indulge in anything that distracts them from real life and avoid the big picture for as long as possible. Uncertainty scares them, so they decide to never feel it again.

But there's another way to live this thing called life. You can find comfort in the uncomfortable, happiness in the present moment, the courage to act by removing all doubts and negative thoughts and emotions.

That's how things are supposed to be anyways. It's just that somewhere down the road we decided to complicate what we do daily, by hiding our feelings, not asking for what we want, keeping ourselves busy with meaningless activities, doing only what gives us instant gratification without thinking long-term, and building a zone of comfort so strong, that it takes some serious character to get out of it.

Some say you need to wait to be ready for a new beginning. I say **it can happen whenever you decide to**, by simply taking your attention from the wrong things, and bringing it back to what matters.

Throughout the book, although each will cover a different field of life that we're quite familiar with, you'll learn a lot about the life-changing practice of letting go. Because to make room for something new and better, you'll need to leave behind something from your current life. By doing it, you'll also free yourself from anything that wasn't taking you in the right direction.

Are you ready to get that started? Any moment other than now will be a bit later. So, let's not postpone the transformation that will open so many new doors for you anymore. Let's make a mindset shift *today*...

***

The subject of the book is social media. And the first chapter that you're about to read will tell you exactly what's wrong with it, and the way we look at it. You'll open your eyes to what's been in front of you the whole time, and get a chance to fix some bad habits and build some better ones.

The following advice and steps are a result of both my personal transformation, but also research and other people's stories who were brave enough to stop the bad influence and welcome more freedom into their life.

The exact process of how you're going to break free is closer to the end, as there are other important steps you need to go through first. It begins with realization. With looking at the bigger picture, being objective, admitting that we've let an outer factor control our thoughts and actions. We need to let it sink in, and that can easily happen by seeing how this has made other people's lives worse.

I'll include plenty of examples for you, including ones from my struggle with social media, to help you see how it has the tendency to become an addictive behavior.

You might have never thought about ditching it fully. I mean, to go completely social media-free. And that's okay. But I believe that by the middle of this book you'll start considering it. Plenty of success stories and studies have proven that a life without any of that part of the digital world is much happier, more peaceful and productive too.

Even if you aren't looking for extreme measures, there's a set of mindful approaches I'll share with you that will turn you into a smart social media user. Then the negative influence on you will be minimum, and you'll move on with your life, while still staying connected.

The next level isn't for everyone, I admit that. But I also thought it wasn't for me either. Until I felt so good when taking a short break of a few days from social networking sites, that I wanted more of that freedom. You too will give that a try and see the benefits. Then you'll be able to decide whether you'll just be taking occasional vacations from your phone, or you want to go further and leave this world behind, together with all that it costs you to be social digitally.

At some point later in the book I get personal and share when I noticed I had a wrong perception of what social media is designed for, and how the first few days of the detox looked like. Not a pretty picture, and it's similar to overcoming other addictions in life. But that only shows how weak we are on its face in the first place, without realizing it.

We often hear that quality is more important than quantity. Well, I'll give you a chance to see that first hand. By not allowing social media to interfere with your personal life and affect your mind, you'll be able to set some limits and still stay connected with those who matter to you the most.

The overall effect of this transformation goes beyond just breaking a bad habit. It's a turning point as it will change your priorities too.

While most people wake up, spend the day and go to bed with a phone in their hand, that has its long-term consequences. And that can be seen only when you put the phone away, rethink what you're doing, and find other ways to be social, that don't include devices.

Your social life will change tremendously. But I promise you this, you'll connect with others in a way that you haven't experienced in a long time. Probably even ever. It's the true nature of relationships - through face-to-face interaction, active listening, showing that you care, and being present.

That sure happened to me. I now know who's most important to me. And that's far from a Facebook list with friends I haven't heard of for years. It's about the real people in your life, the ones you want around, and the ones worth your time and attention. The rest is clutter and only clouds your judgment. So, one positive side of stopping social media is that you'll strengthen your relationships with loved ones and will remove toxic and unimportant people from your life.

The how to's and checklists provided later in the book will be of great assistance if you follow them as you read. Keep your eyes open for the life lessons, as each new beginning brings a ton of these.

I'll now walk you through all that social media is doing to your precious mind, and how that affects all other areas of your life. Once you're aware of the truth, you won't ignore it anymore and will need to do something about it if you're looking to improve the quality of your life.

Then, I'll move onto the tips and steps to bring mindfulness to your life. It usually comes by letting go of anything unnecessary and focusing on what's in front of us in the present moment, and that which is worthy of our attention.

Social media is just wrong, especially in the way we use it these days. So, let me share with you how it might just be the only obstacle to a better life that you need to remove, to finally see progress in any endeavor.

Part 1

The Social Media Effect

With this book, I want to tackle the subject of social media.

I want to show you how it's affecting your life in negative ways. How it's become a disease and has changed today's world in a direction we never desired to go in. How your attention is being sold and the reason for that is in your hands every day. How your behavior is dictated without you realizing, and how your relationships are becoming more and more meaningless.

You have the ability to **choose what you focus on.** And one of the main principles of success is that if you focus on the right things, you'll get them. It's just a matter of time.

Unfortunately, with social media in your life, that's not an option.

In the following chapters, I'll try to reveal the truth about it. The truth which you might not like, as you never had to discuss it openly. But that doesn't make it less harmful.

After that, I'll share with you a practical solution, and depending on the role social media plays in your life, you'll have 2 paths to take.

9

The first is not that extreme and is for those who didn't rely on social networking 24/7 in the first place. I'll show how to be more mindful towards using it, how to set some limits so that you can have more freedom in your life, and how to keep in touch (which is the initial purpose of the existence of social media).

With such small changes, you'll instantly feel better and will start using your time more effectively.

The second solution I'll offer is for those who are quite unhappy with their current life and feel like they haven't seen progress in any areas for years now. Well, you need all your attention back to turn your life around. And social media has no place there.

That's why I'll offer you a plan, including the exact steps you should take to break the habit of using social media sites for hours daily. You'll also get an idea of what life without this toxic practice looks like, and will learn how to stay consistent.

Ready or not, here we go.

Let's begin with the real face of social media and the effect it has on our mind and - ultimately - whole life.

How It Messes with Our Brains

We first need to open our eyes to how exactly social media is affecting our brain.

I'm sure you consider yourself an individual. We all are, after all, as we live in a free world. Or so we think.

Social media is messing with our ability to make decisions, to think independently, to have self-control, and to express ourselves. Let's tackle each of these separately.

Decisions

Each moment of life presents to us multiple choices. Of course, as time is limited, we can do just one thing at a time, be at one place, and engage our minds in one activity.

But by constantly checking our feeds on some social media channels, we've somehow let them be part of our decision-making process.

It might look like a good thing if you go to a restaurant because you saw many friends recommend it on Facebook. Or when you made

11

a purchase because of what an Instagram influencer said about a brand. One week you liked a page because someone invited you and from then on you started being exposed to their messages too. Then, you read a scary tweet about how something we all do daily might be harmful and started making plans on how to break the habit without doing your own research.

These are the tiny ways in which we're influenced at any moment. By the big corporations, by media, by society, and even by our closest friends, simply because they've fallen into the social media trap before us.

The big picture, however, looks completely different. A few years after starting to use social media, a teenager might have a completely new personality and aspirations solely due to the exact channels they are using. An adult might feel dissatisfied with their life and even depressed, even though things looked good before the smartphone started being the most used gadget.

You stop thinking independently.

What happens next is someone else is thinking on your behalf, making choices and telling you how to live your life. But because you're less mindful now, and still see movement, you allow yourself to think you're in control and blame life itself or others for what doesn't go according to your plan.

But it's not them. It's the many outer factors that take your attention and strategically bring it to what's profitable for them. And social media is one of the strongest powers of this generation, that's working against us if we don't start using it wisely.

Turns out, <u>peer pressure</u> is even more big of a deal on social networks, than it is in real life. So, a parent can no longer be calm knowing their kid has good friends and environment, simply because all the bad influences get to its head right in front of the screen, before bed, during school breaks, or at any other moment of the day. That begins the moment you buy it a smartphone without setting some limits.

We lose self-control.

It's easy to slip back into some routines without realizing.

That could be checking Facebook first thing in the morning, while still in bed. The first thoughts we feed our mind with, though, are crucial to what mood we'll be in for the day. Ultimately, how we start our days shapes who we become and what our life looks like.

If each new day begins by scrolling down a feed just because it's something you're used to and do effortlessly, then you end up watching a video or a few without wanting to. You see an old relative inviting you to play a game, someone from college posting details about their life that they could have kept for themselves, another guy you barely know sharing photos from their holiday, and much more.

Does it feel right to let these people in your head, overwhelm yourself with that unnecessary information, and even let your brain start comparing your situation with theirs? No. That's time-wasting and harmful for many reasons.

The point is, by being involved in social media when your brain is most susceptible, you're losing control over your decisions, goals and independent thinking. You might have forgotten how it was before, but you felt much more liberated when social media wasn't a daily thing.

Its Direct Influence on Our Happiness Revealed

Moving onto our level of happiness. Another thing we truly care about and which we'd like to increase one way or another.

Well, a simple formula will be to follow the action steps given later in this book. Why? Because your social media habits are directly related to being unhappy.

For a start, there's the comparing we just mentioned. Regardless of how okay with yourself you are, and even though you might have goals and are eager to achieve them, too many posts of a particular type will make you rethink all that and ask yourself if you're even happy at all.

There's some social media content that is unhealthy to consume. That's the body images of people who seem perfect in every possible way. When the whole Internet is talking about them, there are at least thousands of comments on their posts and your friends are even re-sharing some of that, you can't help but wonder if that's how everyone should be.

And even those most are celebrities and you realize pretty well the photos are edited and you can't get to these people's level and don't even need to, <u>it's proven</u> that the more you look at something, the more you start seeking similarities.

What comes next is noticing all the things you don't have. Thinking how far from that image you are and guessing you'll never get these. Asking yourself if that's fair, and lowering your self-esteem even more. You then go to work and don't feel motivated to do your job. You buy new things to feel good or work out regularly, and still feel like a whole world is separating you from looking like anyone else online.

But there's more to that. And you don't need to be an active social media user for such photos and posts to show up in front of you. They are simply everywhere.

Looking at digital influencers, often at the beach or another luxurious destination in the background, sipping cocktails, or seeing them smiling with their families, shopping, looking good and confident, you realize that you don't have any of that. Or at least not in the same way.

You not just start comparing but also focusing on what's missing in your life. Over time, you feel a void inside, that was never there before.

But here's the thing.

This void is imaginary. It came to be because you let your guard down and allowed something to influence your brain. It turned out to be a well-thought-out tool for changing your whole life, but without your role in it.

It's important to set some time aside and analyze this feeling of emptiness when it occurs again. That might be after ending up checking out your Instagram feed again, or visiting a page that you think inspires you. Or when you accidentally click on a photo and look at the comments, then click on a person's name to see more, and get lost in things you never wanted to see in the first place.

In the next chapter of the book, we'll talk about mindfulness in the era of digital clutter. I believe what you read there will make you more peaceful and let you breathe freely again, as you'll learn to let go of the need for social media and will turn to other things that are more real than this.

But before that, you should assess your current situation.

Take a piece of paper and start jotting down what comes to mind. Invest 5-10 minutes in this simple practice, and know it can be the foundation of the best change you've made in a long time.

You need to be honest with yourself and say things the way they are. Because no one else will do it for you. It's your life and attention we're talking about now, and nothing else matters. So, empty your mind, forget about what your friends might say if you don't message them that often, or that you'll miss seeing certain people's posts daily, or that you have no idea what else to do in the morning instead of grabbing your phone.

You'll see solutions to all these later. For now, just write your soul out and state what your social media behavior looks like, how it might be hurting you, and why you'd like to do less of it. Also, add what new things you'd like to do with your time, or projects to start, or goals to reach, or lifestyle changes to make. That will keep you pumped up, and make you see social media for what they really are - an obstacle to anything else you could be doing.

Information Overload and FOMO

What makes the social media effect even stronger and more personal, is that all our friends are there, and we feel like we're missing out.

Guess what? In any minute there are 347,222 tweets, 31.25 million messages are sent on Facebook, 48,611 photos posted on Instagram, and 300 hours of video uploaded on YouTube. (Source)

These shocking numbers are what the active social media user has to live with daily, knowing how much he's missing out. That's insane, but it also leads to real conditions called information overload and the fear of missing out.

Information overload is that feeling you get after you've logged into one of your accounts just to text someone. But 30 minutes later realized you had scrolled enough feeds and had enough.

It's when you message a dear friend on WhatsApp, but then someone else sends a picture of what he's doing now, and you need to respond. After which it would be rude not to say 'Hey!' to another good friend, or even catch up with the group chats.

You end up being overwhelmed with all the new images and facts and thoughts that enter your mind daily. It's why you can't fall asleep easily if you use your phone in bed. It's why you can't do focused work for long periods of time, and why you need so much time to remember what you did last.

You don't own your attention if your days go like that.

Then, there's the fear of missing out or FOMO. It's something we choose to live with. And until we cut that bad behavior, we'll always be unhappy with what we have, no matter how much it's improving.

The meal you just cooked might seem tasty, but somehow your appetite is lost when you see what some stay-at-home mums do in their free time and post it on Pinterest. Your partner might be the kindest person and the perfect fit for you, but then there will be the couple posting images of their dates, gifts or vacations that look as if it's a dream come true.

But the real fear comes when you truly grasp what more is going on at the same moment. So, if you travel to Spain this summer, and open any social media account, you'll see how others are having fun in all other European resorts. Then, the beach in front of you won't seem that good knowing there are many others better than it.

There are so many examples of that in daily life. And they don't need to be big, such as what event you're currently missing out by being somewhere else. But it's also when you read a post online and are then referred to tens of others on the very same topic. Suddenly, you feel like you know nothing about the subject and want to consume them all. You become anxious, forget about the topic itself, and focus on what else might be out there that needs to be read and understood. You see how limited your time and abilities are, and feel bad about it.

FOMO is one of the main reasons why people join other social media platforms. You'll constantly be prompted to get on Instagram and that can happen with a few clicks once you're on Facebook. You'll be notified when your friends are there, and when they post their first story or photo. All that makes you feel like you're left behind. So you join. You post. You then want more followers. Start using hashtags. Start receiving messages on yet another channel. And add that to your social media rituals that happen a few times daily, which makes the time spent in such activities even longer.

So, less attention for anything else, such as spending time with family, learning things, being outside, having hobbies, reading, planning your future, or just enjoying the silence and relaxing.

These 2 conditions that are a result of the digital world we live in, are something we started experiencing just recently. So, it's safe to say we can remind ourselves of life before social media and find the mental toughness to get over this.

Now, the good news. You can easily take all your happy thoughts, confidence, independence and freedom of choice back, with a few changes on how you go about social media consumption. But before that, there's one last point we should make about the social media effect on us.

When It Becomes an Obsession

Social networking addiction is a real thing. Scarier than information overload and FOMO, for sure. And although it doesn't mean you are or will soon get addicted, even doing it to some extent has its consequences. You'll now learn why social media can sometimes feel better than real life communication. It's important to know exactly what causes social media to feel more comfortable than reality. We can easily leave person-to-person interaction to use our phones and have the imaginary freedom of saying what we want whenever we want it.

To be addicted to something like social media is to crave it. To wake up with that in mind and go to bed with it. To engage your mind in it any minute you're awake, and to leave behind your relationships with those you meet daily.

Here are some examples of excessive use of social networking sites.

There was this guy who fell for online dating so much, that it became his zone of comfort. He boosted his confidence, became a better communicator, knew what works and what doesn't. Even kept interacting with girls for weeks and grabbed their attention with every word, while still playing it casual. But he never went on a real date.

That's because when you meet someone in person, you don't have a screen between you two and that makes you vulnerable. It's because you don't always look your best and can't choose a 'profile picture' that suits your mood. Because you'll be asked questions you won't expect, and wouldn't have the time to pretend like you're not on the phone and think of the best possible answer before replying. So, your image can be ruined, although it was never the real you in the first place.

But when used right, social media can be a good thing. Online dating really leads to meeting the right fit for you and starting something meaningful. But it's just a tool to find that someone and take him or her out. It's the channel you use to get to that real-world interaction as soon as possible. If you skip that and put it off for as long as you can, you form a fake connection that can't survive outside of the digital world.

Moving onto another example.

You might be laughing at those posting pictures of every meal they have or every place they check into and are okay with yourself doing it just every now and then when there's a special occasion. But once you knew what was going on in these people's heads, you would feel bad for them.

Anxiety has many faces, as you might know. And social media networking is often contributing to that. It brings unnecessary and fake desires and needs. The more you give in to following the crowd - in this case, posting updates for everything you do, showing you're actually doing a lot - the more you need to keep this going. Your life soon becomes a struggle as you eventually go through a more boring period in your life, and others will immediately notice the fact that you haven't been to a restaurant in a few weeks.

Women, once they start making selfies and maybe adding a quote here and there, need to look good 24/7. The appearance and personality on social media need to be consistent, otherwise, your reputation worsens.

That might sound like nothing you'd do, but even the small signs (the initial stage of addiction) are something to be concerned about. Unhealthy behaviors tend to escalate quickly. Without monitoring this, you can fall into a deep hole.

I'm bringing your attention to the chance of getting obsessed with social media now, to show you why setting limits will save you from this. We'll talk about that in the next chapter. But before that, let's see the science-backed aspects of social media addiction, and the symptoms that can be seen in daily life.

What Science Says

Researchers have found that social media - or using Facebook and Twitter in particular - is more addictive than cigarettes and alcohol.

Another thing we might need to keep in mind is a study that found out Facebook and Internet addiction in general, activate the same parts of the brain as cocaine. Scientists state using Facebook is perceived by the mind as any other important event during the day. What's more, the moment we open it, we get the satisfaction of being rewarded. So, it's no wonder we need to repeat that behavior as many times as we can per day.

But in that same research, candidates responded more quickly to an image of Facebook than to one of a road sign. Which shows us our brain is more susceptible to social media than to reacting instantly when we need to, such as when driving a car and seeing a Stop sign. Or that people are better prepared to answer a message on their phones when hearing the familiar noise of Messenger, than to the traffic in front of them.

That's not a guess, though. You might not have gotten this far as to care more about your phone than the other cars on the road, but it's proven that most car accidents are due to distractions like that. To be more precise, researchers checked the phones of the drivers that took part in an accident and found that more than 50% of them were on their phones at the time of the event.

While other studies proved that what people crave the most during the day are sleep and sex. However, on top of that comes the urge to check and update social media. Seems like this is what we give in to the most.

And here's how resisting temptations works: you wake up with a ton of willpower in the morning and say 'no' to temptations and distractions for a few hours while getting ready for the day and getting to school or work. You have control for some time, although the urges are almost always in your mind. You reject each, but every next time it's harder. Your willpower is decreasing (it's a finite resource) and at some point, you know you'll need to grab your phone and give it 15-30 minutes. You might do it just for 3-5-minute sessions the first few times, but that will just give you the feeling of comfort and being social. These feel familiar, so your mind wants its next dose, and in a bigger amount.

The longer you keep it up, the better. But as the day goes by, your self-control is also disappearing. You start making excuses to yourself as to why you need social media. That might be things like having to reply to your friends cause they might get offended, or to check somebody's feed as there was something important he was going through and you need to see if he's okay (even without personally reaching out to him), to see what's posted on your favorite pages, to check updates in the fields you're following, to see recent likes on your last few posts, to answer some comments, to upload a nice photo you made yesterday, to check out that new filter Snapchat just released, to see the latest funny videos your friends tagged you in, and more.

It begins with one scroll, one message, one look. But it evokes all emotions in your brain and activates processes for the wrong reasons.

Social media has become the most dangerous type of addiction for the next generations, as kids use technology the moment they develop cognitive skills.

Social Media Addiction Symptoms

The first one would be grabbing your phone first thing in the morning. Not because it's near you and you just hit snooze, but because you do open Facebook and scroll down the feed, consuming any type of content that comes your way without thinking about it. That's before you've left the bed, or even let your mind become alert and welcome the new day. By doing this, you're basically telling the brain that social media matters the most. You give it its dose of updates and attention before the day has started, and you'll be feeding it with it every hour or so until the evening.

You often find yourself looking at your phone for a long time without taking your eyes off it while walking or doing something else that requires your attention elsewhere.

You're often on the verge of missing your stop when using public transport, or being late for work or a meeting, as you've lost track of time because of your smartphone and all that's going on online.

When you haven't received new friend requests or follows, or enough attention on your latest posts or comments, or when someone hasn't seen your message for more than a day, you feel something that resembles loneliness. And that's nothing surprising. Because while in the past the size of your social circle was the reason whether or not you feel lonely and miss enough communication and connectedness, now it's the popularity on social media, or the lack of it, that replaces this. Meaning, some people who aren't doing well in real life, but who get attention on social media (be it by making videos and getting many views, being followed by new people daily due to funny statements they make, or receiving many messages), are considered popular. Unfortunately, that does play a role and they are likely to skip any face-to-face interaction as it just won't give them what their social media personality is giving them. So, they are more likely to spend a ton of time daily on their smartphones, keeping their fans entertained and feeling great about it.

That is yet another symptom of addiction, as it takes over one of the most important aspects of your life - socializing with real human beings. And because the same effect can never be reached, you might soon start seeing signs of depression. The lack of being tapped on the shoulder, handshaking a new friend of a friend, using body language to open up to someone while chatting, and more - without all this you can't live a fulfilling life.

The next stage of this is social anxiety. When you don't feel comfortable in public, prefer to chat with somebody rather than meet them, and when you feel like checking your phone when you are out with friends.

What's more, social media users who get obsessed with this, fear their battery going dead. Luckily, there are enough tools these days to keep it charged 24/7, and anywhere you go.

You're also addicted if you sometimes do new activities like jogging, taking a walk, meeting an old friend and waiting for him at the cafe, but not leaving your phone at any free second. It makes you feel like at home, even though you're not in a familiar environment.

A big part of personal growth is defining how your zone of comfort looks and finding ways to break free from it. That usually happens by trying new stuff, doing things you're afraid of and challenging yourself by consciously putting yourself in new (possibly uncomfortable) situations. But with a phone in your hand, your comfort zone also becomes mobile and it's just a locked screen away. The only way out is to ditch your phone for certain times of the day, to limit social media usage, build new habits, or completely unplug for some time to breathe freely and live life.

There are more symptoms of social media networking obsession that you might have noticed or experienced yourself.

Some people truly love their phone and spend most of their time together with it. I mean, depending on what else they have to do, they might hold it for hours in a row. It feels nice to know it's in your hand and to be able to respond to a new message or check notifications the moment you receive them.

When on holiday or just for drinks with friends on a sunny day, most people post so many updates that you start wondering whether they participate in the talk with the people present in the situation or enjoy the view in front of them at all.

Things are getting in the addiction direction also when you start hearing important news on social media first. Such as a celebrity who died, a new terrorist attack, a local event you didn't know about, a political scandal, or even what's going to happen on the next episode of your favorite show.

When using social media with limits, though, it can serve as an information source and be practical if you only open up networks with that in mind, check the news in the right places, and leave. But in this case, it means learning things from someone you barely know and seeing his ridiculous opinion on it, which is something you didn't really need. It means having a lot in your mind that doesn't need to be there, and which takes your attention during the day away from your work and goals.

Social media addicts can also be recognized by the language they are using. Previous generations won't understand a word. As you might hear things like 'hashtag', 'tweet', 'whatsapp me', 'swiping left', 'lol', and more.

Social media is changing our language, and that makes the digital world part of real-life communication. Eventually, it takes over and we feel like it's enough to just message someone every now and then.

This is also causing restlessness. That's when you feel nervous and somehow empty if you haven't checked your phone for some time, and are now dying to interrupt your current activity - whatever that is - and just get to it and see what you've missed.

The question that remains is, once inside the social media effect trap, how does one get out safely?

What's the Solution?

The solution comes in many forms that when combined, lead to the ultimate free mind, allowing you to take any direction in life and see progress soon.

With the self-assessment exercise, you must have done earlier, you get a clear understanding of what's going on. That brings your attention to the present moment for a while and you feel like you got this, or at least can do more about it to handle the issue.

The present moment is all we have. It's real life and the only place we should be at. That means not thinking about the past, not being worried about the future, and not using social media to get attention or be entertained with other people's lives. Mindfulness is about acknowledging you're leading astray, and peacefully getting back here, enjoying what is around you, accepting it, letting go of any rush or comparing or discomfort.

There are a few important elements connected to mindfulness and we'll tackle each one separately in the following chapter. That will slowly lead to so much more space in your mind, that you'll be able to fill with positive thoughts and influences.

You'll become stronger as a result, and each next decision or action you take will contribute to your courage. You'll get out of your comfort zone effortlessly if you do it all slowly, one step at a time.

What matters too, is looking at this whole transformation as a good thing. Don't feel intimidated by the time it might take. Don't be scared of not knowing where to start. You'll be given a plan in this book and can personalize it based on your lifestyle and interests.

And while the destination is what makes the journey complete, you need to understand that the actual process is not just exciting, but also beautiful and a must on your path to self-improvement and success.

Smile now for what's awaiting. New beginnings are challenging, but the fact that you're doing something about your future itself is motivating and even inspiring for others around you.

I made that shift and was particularly invested in breaking the social media pattern. That led to more opportunities and independence than I ever knew existed.

So, you've got a reason to be proud of yourself already if you made the first step of writing down the good, the bad and the ugly in your relationship with social media.

As unpleasant as it might be, without this step you can't continue. But even this little action makes your 10 minutes of writing and musing much better spent than anyone else attached to their screen checking out other people's profiles.

I'm excited for you too as I know how much you'll change if you disconnect and start paying attention to more meaningful things.

Now, let's talk about setting some limits and saying 'no' to social media a bit more often.

Part 2

The Mindful User

Now you know why social media is bad for us all, and where it goes wrong when we start using it daily. But that doesn't mean it has nothing practical in it. There are some meaningful ways in which we can benefit from it, that weren't available decades ago.

If you don't overdo it, and set some limits and follow the mindful practices described later in this chapter, you will be able to do all of this, without being overwhelmed or getting addicted or feeling lonely, depressed or distracted:

1. Keeping in touch with friends.

It's easy, it's fast, it's convenient. Sometimes, it can be the reason why you are still friends with somebody, but if there are still topics to talk about, it's all good. It's not always necessary to leave what you're doing and go meet a friend, especially if you two live in different cities. But a single message asking about their day can be the reason why you are still in each other's lives. Although digital, that's still communication and connection and reminds us we have people we care about.

2. Connecting with the world.

It still amazes me how much social media can offer and that it takes a single click of a button (to search a hashtag, for instance), to find like-minded people from all corners of the world. Then, in a few seconds, you can connect with them in a friendly way and see if they respond. You can then discuss your topic of interest, share ideas, become friends, form a community with others involved in the same field, and more. All that costs nothing but can make a big difference in your life, regardless of what you're passionate about.

3. Inspiration in your pocket.

I know some people who drag themselves to the gym and eat healthy just because they read enough motivational quotes and follow the right online personalities. Each post on these profiles aims to inspire the followers. It could be the prepped meals for the weak of a fitness instructor. Or the new exercise a fit girl is trying that is also challenging for her regardless of her experience. Not to mention the many before and after pics, we can find everywhere online. That kind of inspiration exists on social media in the most realistic way possible. In the past that could have been magazines, but the people on the covers never looked like they are from this world, or happy for that matter.

Then there are the videos. Aspiring entrepreneurs need a 30-second YouTube session to get pumped up and get to work on their next online business idea. Even if no one in their life supports them, if they are far from being self-employed and stuck in a day job, they just need to hear it from someone else who's been there and who's escaped that reality, to enter the entrepreneurial world.

In such ways, social media is encouraging us to be our best. If we only choose the right content to consume, the genuine people who aren't in it for the money, and avoid anything other than this.

4. Career advancement.

Job networking is a real thing. It might mean a student who's got an online presence can be found by a potential employer. Or someone wants to enter a new field and builds connections over time on social networks for professionals such as LinkedIn.

You no longer need to collect degrees, do tens of internships, attend interviews, deal with competition, etc.

It's about initiative. If you're truly determined and believe you have qualities that can contribute to somebody's business, then just go ahead and take a few actions online to prove it. I've heard plenty of stories about people who just emailed or messaged an influencer with an offer they couldn't refuse, offered to work for them for free so they can learn from them, and who did such a good job that later became their employees and changed their career trajectory.

5. Research and information.

Information is powerful, and it's all easily accessible. When looking for a job, learn anything you can about the company and the field.

You'll be prepared for any question this way, and can even form your opinion on some important matters in the field that you can later share with superiors and show you know a thing or two.

And you no longer need to just browse the Web. It's all on social media. Check out the company page on different channels and scroll down. See their latest updates, but also go back to company events from last year. You'll get a feeling of their values and what they expect from anyone joining the team.

6. Real-time updates.

Communication travels fast on social media. In fact, you can accidentally see a status about something happening 2 streets from you. Maybe even watch a live video. At the same time, in the comments appearing at any minute, depending on how popular the person is and how much attention this update is getting, you can see people from other places, or those nearby, sharing information related to the case. That's better than the news and can save a life sometimes.

What's more, it's getting more and more common to share a post about a missing person and encourage your friends living in the same area to re-share. Because of that, you increase the chances of him being found.

The same goes for warnings about something unexpected.

Keeping these in mind, we'll now proceed to the action part. I want to give you some practical tips on how to use social media in new, more conscious ways so that you can make the most of this. Then, the balance will be reached. In this case, it means not turning your phone into a distraction and social media into a useless, tempting aspect of your life that's with you at any moment of the day. But, instead, using it wisely, with limits, and to do the real things that are helping you and making life easier and better.

Quality over Quantity

The problem with social media is that it's just too much. The chats heads, the notifications, the posts of friends you see in your feed, the news that pop up, the people on your list, the comments everywhere. You get lost in all this and your mind can't choose what to focus on. So, it just does it all on autopilot, letting you feed it with whatever's in front of you.

Let's say 'No'. But not to social media in general. That you can do in the next chapter if you're serious about changing the direction you've taken in life and need to focus on the absolute essentials to reach your goals. For now, let's limit our usage and change our approach. The main thing between all that you're about to read now, is that you'll prefer quality.

That means **not using all channels**. It takes too much time and that leads to more information, people and updates coming your way at any minute.

It means **having fewer followers and friends** in your list or numbers in your phone. You don't need too many, so let's leave only the ones you communicate with regularly, or even every now and then.

And what about the things you've subscribed to, have liked in the past, or are following without knowing? You see the updates of these people and brands constantly, and they engage your brain when you need to be focused on other things.

That's why it's time to set some limits. To say no to all that isn't essential, so you can make room for what matters and pay enough attention to it without going crazy.

Social Media Decluttering

We can call that social media decluttering.

Decluttering is closely related to minimalism, which is the art of removing anything that shouldn't be there, and keeping only what matters. That's popular with design and fashion, but also for personal qualities, productivity and time management (removing all tasks and activities that don't bring you progress, and working more on the rest), etc.

There's clutter if you don't remove something, and that's especially true for social networking.

How many times did you end up chatting with an old friend just because he saw a post of yours, but there isn't really something you have to discuss? How often do you end up watching a video or clicking on a link just because it appeared on your timeline?

If you calculate all the time you waste weekly, you'd be surprised to learn what a big chunk of it social media is consuming. Just imagine what else you could do with that same amount of precious time!

Consider this your spring cleaning session. You know how it feels when you get rid of some old belongings, or finally, organize the chaos on your desk, or sell some old stuff and don't buy anything new.

That's like a therapy. It's good for the mental health too, and you feel positive about it. The reason for this is we have the tendency to get attached to almost anything. And when we choose the minimalist approach - to be ruthless and remove anything that doesn't mean a lot to us - we feel freedom like no other thing can give us.

That's exactly what I did with my social media usage, and why I want you to do the same. The amount of time you get back is surprising, but so is the clarity you gain, the creative energy that comes back to you, the peace of mind in the mornings and evenings when you're okay with not checking your phone. The lack of rush is also a benefit of decluttering.

Believe it or not, you too have some attachment in your relationship with social media. If something's such a big part of your day and engages your mind that often, it surely costs you emotions, you have expectations, it brings you comfort, and so on. Most of these are negative and you end up relying on this to make you feel good. Such influences should be under our control, though. And that's where setting some limits to social networking comes.

We'll now talk about the exact ways in which you can block the negative social media impact on you, and you'll learn about some awesome practices of the mindful user that you can adopt. They will make you more peaceful and your days will be more productive and filled with energy. Your mind will be clearer, and your soul happier due to these little changes.

So, how do we set these limits to something so addictive?

By being aware of its bad influence and keeping in mind all the information of the previous chapter.

By reminding ourselves this is not where our attention is supposed to be and that there are better things to invest it in.

By being determined to take back control of our mind and life.

By choosing less (in terms of information, channels, and people) but realizing it leads to more (deeper relationships with the right people, reading only what matters and can make a difference in our lives, and using social media only for its benefits).

Are you ready to become conscious about socializing online?

Conscious Ways to Use Social Media

Have intentions.

Let's begin with something simple, but which can be a turning point in for your relationship with social media. Whenever you open it, have a reason for that.

In the beginning, you'll end up opening apps or browsing feeds without realizing. It takes seconds to unlock your phone and be thrown into the ocean of information. Your mind is inside the digital world already, it becomes harder to get your eyes off it, you are taken to the next notification, the next update, the next message. Until it's been 20 minutes, and you're procrastinating.

Even when you set intentions for using it, this scenario will still happen often. And that's alright. The process is slow, but it's the foundation of your life without addiction to any gadget or channel.

What does it mean to have intentions when it comes to online communication? Well, there's a need you want to meet every time you do something. The same goes for logging in to Facebook, opening Twitter or posting on Instagram. It's usually on a subconscious level, but you can dig a bit and find it out. Once it's defined, you can rationalize and decide whether the action is worth your time.

Although there will be excuses your mind will come up with as to why there is indeed a reason to be on social media for at least 5 minutes (as it's used to that), this little exercise is a good start. It will soon become a habit. You'll automatically stop and take a moment to analyze why you're doing what you're about to do before getting online. You'll take a few seconds to think it through. And most often this little break is a good enough barrier to proceeding with the action and wasting the next 10 minutes in pointless digital behavior.

The moment you stop the automatic action, done without thinking, of answering a message or seeing what's new on your favorite platform, is the moment you take back control of your attention. You then ask yourself what's going on and can recognize the signs of addiction. That will make you cut the usage of social sites in half. You'll also build willpower as that approach can be applied to any other bad habit you're struggling with breaking.

Over time, you'll also remember the many times you used social media without intention. Nothing good came out of it, no doubt about that.

I do remember what was going on in my brain back in the days when I allowed social media to affect me in more ways than I wanted. Although not the biggest fan of technology in general, I'd grab my phone for something, and instead just open Facebook, see what's on top, then scroll down for a bit, then maybe click on the name of someone posting an item that grabbed my attention and start thinking how I know him and what's been going on with him since then.

That's a vicious cycle. Life is much easier when you say 'stop' before you've fallen into the trap of the latest updates. Because that's the thing about real-time information - it never stops.

So, from now on, analyze your intention before entering the social media world. Ultimately, that's how we should go about any other activity in our lives.

Organize your day well.

One of the reasons why we become frequent social media users is because we find ourselves with free time quite often during the day. That might be due to lack of good time management and organizational skills. So, if we fix these, then we'll need to avoid the bad phone habits much less and thus save our willpower for more important things.

For instance, grabbing your phone first thing in the morning means you haven't really planned out the early hours of your day so you've got time to waste. But it makes you lazy and you barely find the motivation to leave the house.

What successful people do instead is create morning routines. These are a set of healthy, positive and productive habits that are meant to set you up for a great day. It usually begins by preparing for your morning the night before.

Keep in mind that the practices in this and the following sections of the chapter can turn your whole life around and get you closer to your goals. Limiting social media usage and having a clear mind are just 2 of the benefits.

If you spend 5 minutes every evening to write down a list of what you need to get done tomorrow, you'll also be able to wake up and get to action. Plan your morning down to the last detail. Leave no free time for distractions. You can still have relaxing activities such as drinking your coffee in silence, stretching, reading something, making breakfast, getting ready for going out, etc. But these too should be written down to become part of your day. Otherwise, there won't be order and it's easy to grab your phone again.

With such a start of the day, you'll have more focus than you usually do. You will check social media later and it will still affect you, but if you get back your mornings, you'll have made a big leap in your personal growth.

Structuring an effective day doesn't end with this. You can do the same with your evenings. They are especially important as it's the time of the day you should get to rest and prepare your mind and body for sleep. Without this, your sleep patterns will be interrupted, and you won't get the rest you need. As a result, you won't wake up fresh and in a great mood tomorrow morning. It's all connected, you see. And ditching your phone in the morning and evening will make you more disciplined and you'll be getting more done during the day.

If you don't know where to start to live a better life and be free of the negative influence of social networking, then do this: plan out tomorrow morning, wake up with a smile on your face and have a pleasant ritual to start the day. That will change the whole picture.

Choose authenticity.

By using social media sites for some time, you start building an online persona. Whether you like it or not, you sometimes end up answering those you don't feel like chatting with. Or posting something because it's a trending topic. Or you add a comment to a post that's getting a lot of attention from your friends. Maybe you join a group because it's suggested to you by someone you like. Or you hit the like button on a picture you don't fancy that much, but which will affect your relationship with that person in a positive way.

Unfortunately, none of that is your real self. You're leading astray from authenticity due to peer pressure, the need for attention, seeking approval, following the crowd, and more. But simply limiting your time on these channels will guarantee you a better, more authentic relationship with your true self.

Pretending to be someone we're not, makes us miserable. We try to answer expectations of people we don't even respect, and end up becoming someone we aren't happy with. Then, we might get attention online, but in reality, we don't even talk or behave this way.

One of the main rules of success is to embrace who you are. You're an individual and have a ton of potential inside. It's waiting to be unleashed. But bad habits like social media, when used in a wrong way, are preventing you from being authentic.

The next time you're about to post something or to take any action on a platform like that, stop and ask yourself if you're doing it because you want to, or due to another factor. Sometimes you might want to be appreciated, grab attention, look cool, start a discussion to see what others will say, do something because everyone else did it, or follow updates in order not to feel left behind. But all that is fake. It's not what you're supposed to be doing with your time. So, let go, and better leave your phone instead of turning into a social media user with no real personality.

There's a way to make the best of both worlds.

You can be authentic, and make the most of social media while being selective and careful with your attention and time.

That means only making a post when there's something you truly want to share with your people online. When there's a topic you're passionate about and you want to bring attention to it. When you're being direct and not leaving anything behind.

Other social media activities, such as leaving a comment, following someone, liking a page or an image, sending a message, accepting a request, will need careful consideration now. Never do it if you don't genuinely feel like doing it.

But when you do take some of these little actions, let that come from the bottom of your heart. It's simple. If you like someone, you tell them. If you think they shared a smart quote, you leave a comment to let them know you dig that. If you aren't interested in a topic, you never like pages or follow people in that niche.

That's how you use social media consciously and let it be a practical and positive thing in your life, instead of a distraction.

Now, let's see what a mindful user really does before, during and after social media-related activities.

Practices of The Mindful User

1. Stop the cycle.

You open your phone, log in one social media channel and spend 5 minutes there. You see enough, nothing exciting seems to be going on now. Then you do the same with 3 more platforms.

But by the time you're done with them, you're anxious to do it all over again. It's like the first action never happened and something new can be happening that you just can't afford to miss. So, you go to Facebook again, maybe engage in a conversation or two, then move onto the next app that's opened.

How long can that continue? And can you recognize the tiny signs of addiction?

Mindfulness is the way out because you will stop before, during or after each action on social media, and ask yourself why you're doing it, whether it's your own intention, or consider the time you're wasting and what else you could have done with your focus. These are powerful little mental habits that will help you stay on the right track.

When you are about to begin the cycle described above, you can refuse to get yourself into this and just go do something else. Ultimately, the goal is to be able to do it every time. But once you're logged in, things escalate quickly, and your mind is already in the ocean of information. So, it's easier to prevent that before it's started, rather than to try and escape earlier once you're in.

The Habit Loop

It all begins with awareness. Now you know how the cycle looks like. But also consider when it usually happens. Think of the moments when you grab your phone and waste half an hour without realizing. You'll find some tendencies. Maybe it's during a work break, or when you're bored, or when you procrastinate, or after a meal, or when you hear the sound of a notification.

This is the so-called habit loop. Something Charles Duhigg explores in his bestseller 'The Power of Habit'. He shares that for everything we do repeatedly (that's what a habit means, after all), there a cue, routine and reward. These elements form the neurological loop that directs any habitual behavior we have. Most of what we do is unhealthy and done unconsciously, simply because we haven't identified the cue and routine, to know what we're doing wrong and where to start when looking for a change.

An example would look like this. The cue is waking up, the routine is reaching for your phone, the reward is feeling a sense of connectedness (even on a digital level).

There are many things we can try to turn around in this scenario. For instance, in order to break the whole morning habit, we should immediately do something else upon waking up. But then the brain wouldn't receive the reward it's used to and will crave it soon again.

The reward can be the comfort social media gives you, or to keep up with what you've missed while sleeping, or to check a group chat, or just feel like you're socializing without really interacting with somebody in particular.

Know why you're doing it. That will help you know what positive feeling you get out of this habit, and you can seek it in other ways.

A way to replace this habit (and all other bad phone habits that we do later in the day), is to go talk to a loved one at home, or to a colleague at work. Then your phone becomes useless and you still get the feeling of being social, which is one of the most important human needs and shouldn't be underestimated.

The cue in this morning scenario is the act of leaving the bed. Obviously, that will always happen. But in other cases, a cue might be the fact that it's Sunday morning, or that you can leave work earlier, or the commercials when watching TV. All these are what provokes you to keep doing the bad habits you're trying to avoid. So, make changes accordingly.

Basically, the solutions Charles Duhigg gives for breaking such habits that have been with us for a long time and which seem unavoidable now, are the following:

Know exactly how your routine looks like - that's what you're trying to avoid. In the example above, it's opening your eyes, grabbing your phone, and then taking the next steps depending on your preferences. Could be answering messages from last night first, then seeing notifications on Facebook, then purposelessly scrolling down the feed and accidentally watching a video or two.

Identify your reward. - know what you're getting out of all this that your brain is happy with and which makes it seek it again.

Replace it. - look for other simple and more meaningful ways to get the same or similar reward (much like talking to a colleague at work instead of chatting with random people, which is far from real communication);

Remove the trigger - that's the cue and it can be the place you're at, the people around you (if everyone's checking their phone at a certain time of the day, you're more likely to do it too), a certain hour of the day, after another thing you do often, etc. Know what it is that provokes the routine and the reward that follows. Try to break this cue or make it less powerful by changing something about it.

Now you know a bit more about how habits are formed and how our brain works when doing something repeatedly. This makes it easier to break the cycle.

2. Fixed times of the day.

Reading this book doesn't mean everyone will limit their social media usage today and become a new person tomorrow. For some, it might take a week to understand the principles, take some decisions, and then start making an actual change. That itself will take 2-4 weeks to be formed as a habit and be done effortlessly.

No rush, though. Slow progress remains forever, and that's what we're trying to achieve here. Now that you know you should organize your whole day in a new, better way to ditch bad habits such as too much social media, it's also worth working with fixed times for doing and not doing things. Here's what I mean.

You can limit social media at certain times of the day, and you can then decide on fixed parts of the day for when you can use it. How awesome is that! Full control over when you're using your phone and when it can't distract you.

Let me give you more specific tips with examples for both situations. Keep in mind that this section of the chapter involves your self-discipline and personal organization, while the next one will offer you some tools to block your access to social media at certain times. Both are worth trying to see what works best for you.

Not using social media at certain times of the day.

Times of the day when you're better off without your phone are these:

- Upon waking up;
- Any time you're bed;
- An hour before bed;
- In your car;
- While walking;
- During a meal;
- When talking to someone face-to-face;
- Waiting in a queue;
- Reading or writing;
- Working out.

Chances are, one of these is something you always do with your phone in hand. And it might look like an innocent way of multitasking, but it's not because the negative influences of social media are still attacking your brain and that affects the rest of your life if done daily.

Don't decide to stop using your phone at all the situations and times of the day listed above, though. That will lead to using all your willpower early on, and being left with an even bigger desire to spend an hour on networking sites.

Choose one to start with and it will help you build the discipline to achieve more with your next small goals, all of which are bringing you closer to the freedom of a life without any social media addiction.

So, don't allow yourself to use your phone in your car tomorrow. Then, put it away from your bed a few days after that so that you can go and get it (a good way to actually wake up with the first alarm, by the way), and that will help you to not be lying with it in hand (which makes it comfortable to just stay like this for a long time even though the day has started).

Another thing you can do is use silent mode while working, or being at an important family event, or when on a date. This way you won't be tempted to see who just texted you or sent you a friend request.

Having set times for social networking.

The next step is to allow yourself to use your phone for anything social-media-related but to do so only at certain times. That can be after you've done your most important work for the day or when having half an hour for chilling after work (but don't multitask by watching TV at the same time as it makes it yet another unconscious period of time).

Do this when there's literally nothing else to do. It's practical if you do it right after another activity has been completed, and you can now engage your brain in a completely different way. That boosts focus and productivity. Because being concentrated on one thing for a long time leads to boredom, lack of motivation to do a good job, desire to procrastinate, etc. So social media, if done with limits and used wisely, can be a good in-between task that helps your mind recharge after a work session.

3. Set deadlines.

To take things further, a mindful online user would also set deadlines. These are proven to make the human brain perform better and we somehow do all that we planned to do in a shorter period. So, let's use the power of deadlines to our advantage, and still have our social networking time but with limits in terms of how long we stay on the phone.

That might mean using it sometime in the morning or during your lunch break (if you're okay with not limiting usage in terms of times of the day but prefer another approach). In such cases, you are free to log in to any channel you want, do whatever you feel like, but know you have a limited amount of time for that.

That's an awesome trick as it makes us skip anything meaningless and just get to the point. It also shows you how much of what you do once logged in is unnecessary.

Of course, you need to take that seriously. You can also find an accountability buddy and share the results with them so that you can be motivated to say only positive things.

4. Limit the number of activities you do on social media.

Here's another thing you can add to your new approach to social networking or even a way to set your first limits before moving onto another step. These are in no particular order so just begin with what feels comfortable.

What if you stop doing some of the things you do on your phone, and just leave the ones that mean something and give you results?

For instance, why bother with ever clicking on a person's name again to see their profile? Set this as your next mini goal for this new beginning you're getting closer to.

Or you can say no to pinning images on Pinterest, checking notifications on Twitter, posting on both Instagram and Facebook when uploading a photo, using Messenger for chats, voice and video calls (it's just too much, pick one).

Once you say no to some of these, your experience on these sites and apps will be lighter and much more enjoyable. You'll be able to respond to everyone who's important and to keep the conversation going, you won't waste too much time, and won't feel like you're missing out on a lot.

Know that not all activities are necessary. Disciplined and productive people know our time and focus are limited, so we need to be selective with what we dedicate them to. Limit your choices, and you'll do what's left with all your attention.

5. Ditch a few platforms today.

Time to say goodbye to all those channels you have a profile on, have posted on back in the days, receive notifications from but don't check them, or joined because of a reason that's not relevant anymore.

Don't just log out. Go there now and delete your profile. Sometimes, it's not easy to find that in the settings. And this is not a coincidence. The creators don't want you to leave their platforms. They might keep sending you reminders and emails to get back again, saying they miss you, reminding you of your last posts or even mentioning who of your Facebook friends are on their site too. Don't let them fool you.

The sites you'll leave today are the ones where you don't have anyone important, with whom you also don't have contact anywhere else. It means, you just decide you don't have time for that and don't want to see alerts from something you've barely used in the last year. It makes sense to delete your profile. By doing this, you're also letting go of what you've posted or seen there. That's great. It gives room for better things.

6. A cute little practice to do before logging in.

If you're a social media user who's already online before even realizing your phone was in your hand, then you'll benefit from this meditative practice.

When it's time for socializing in the digital world, or you receive a message and can't wait to see it, stop before getting your phone, take a few deep breaths. That's all you need to get back to the present moment.

Then, remind yourself what you're about to do now, acknowledge the fact it's not the best use of your time, define your intention, and say what you will do exactly. This gives you a plan to follow and you're less likely to get too distracted with random things.

If you're ready for more mindfulness, you can also stop before opening the chat head or clicking the app icon. You have some expectations in your mind now, be it about who texted you, how many new things you'll see, whether you've got comments on your latest post, or else. Notice each of these and let go of that. Expectations are meaningless. They lead to disappointment. The best use of social media is to enter it with a clear mind and just go with the flow, for a short time, and then get back to reality.

There's another step to that too. It's what you can do after you open the app and have already seen a notification, message, or post in your feed. Again, you can take a break for a few seconds, breathe deeply, and see how you just felt. That's a fantastic approach to understanding how social media affects your emotions and recognizing which types of posts, or which exact people you chat with for that matter, are causing you negative feelings.

It's hard to admit you've had a sense of jealousy after seeing somebody's picture, for instance. But better just let it out now and let go, instead of keeping it inside.

This mindful practice will make you feel better about yourself too, you'll finally feel in control of your actions and thoughts, and will then be able to make a change that lasts forever.

7. Recognize what's not real.

There's this little test you can try, each time you're online and ready to get back to your old habits. Let's call it the 'Is It Real?' test.

It's about making a difference between what's a true form of communication, and what's not.

Remember the benefits of social media we mentioned at the beginning of this chapter? Well, you can only experience them if you use it in a meaningful way. And that means to keep in touch with dear friends, to get only the information you need, to be inspired by the right sources, etc.

To make sure you don't do anything other than that on your phone, ask yourself if it's real or not before hitting a button. You'll be surprised how many times a certain activity has no actual purpose. So, it doesn't make sense to complete the action once you're aware of this.

8. Stop seeking validation.

Imagine this common scenario: somebody posts a picture of them dressed sharply at a nice restaurant, or event. For a start, this action is basically saying 'Look at me. I'm here and look good, and you aren't and don't.' That's harmful to the self-esteem of the creator and the consumer of this type of content, by the way.

But it gets worse if you let it affect you in a way where you seek validation and need to post something similar to show others in your friends list that you're having a good time too. That's fake, brings pressure to one's life, and makes everyone feel bad at the end of the day.

Being on the beach and taking a picture of your legs, while getting the beer, sea, and sand in it too, is something we see too often. And if we are stuck in the office at the same time, we immediately feel not just upset, but truly miserable. If that happens every day for a month, imagine how it can ruin any determination you have to change your life and do better.

To never use social media for bragging again, or to seek validation, ask this simple question before uploading a photo or tagging yourself in a location you're visiting for the first time:

Am I providing value with this?

Because if you aren't, then there's simply no point in sharing that part of your day with anyone you know in the digital world, and you're better off getting back to the present moment and experiencing it and having a good time.

9. Know when to put the phone away.

Finally, the mindful online user likes to take a break once he's posted or sent a message. Meaning, you did something on social media, so leave the phone away. It's enough for now. You want this in small doses if you aim to have limits.

But what most people do instead is eagerly await responses, comments, and likes on their last photo, notifications coming from what they just shared, or else. That causes anxiety and you can stay online for hours trying to check the newest reactions you get the moment they come in.

Stop right there. That doesn't matter. You've said what you had to, now it's time to walk away. That's another little way to let go of the pressure and overwhelming feelings, and to continue with your other activities for the day. The next time you go online, you'll see it all. And will then respond quickly and take another break. I believe this will make your time spent on social media sites much easier and more pleasant.

10. Do one thing at a time.

One of the main characteristics of someone who's aware of their actions at any moment of the day, is that he's only doing one thing and is fully invested in it. Multitasking kills focus and productivity, and on social media, it means even more tension and information overload.

Limit the things you're doing there at the same time. Why chat with 5 people? You easily forget what you just said, read their responses quickly and miss the point, it takes you longer to take a decision and schedule a meeting or just finish a discussion. So, it becomes a burden. But to use the platform wisely, chat or talk to one person at a time. It's like you're face to face but separated by a screen.

The same goes for having more than one app opened. It makes you eager to switch between them, and you don't have a single second to process what you just saw or read.

Instead, take it easy by doing one thing at a time. If you're reading a status, do it slowly, forget about anything else. If you're talking to someone, don't check notifications at the same time, listen to that person and respond accordingly. It's okay to wait a few seconds between answers. Here's the moment to just enjoy the conversation that's going on instead of killing time by logging in to another site.

So, these are the practices of the mindful user. Sounds great, right? It might also seem like a lot of work, but as I said, you don't need to get it done all at once. It's a process of social media decluttering and all processes happen slowly over time.

Go through the 10 points above again. Choose one, to begin with. Think of ways to implement it in your daily life over the next few days. Don't forget to track the results too. And by results, I mean everything that happens in your mind when you're about to use social media, the actual things you use your phone for, how long it takes, and how you feel after that.

That itself is a journey to self-realization. It can help you understand your motives, desires, expectations, and doubts. That is later used for taking your personal development to the next level.

Now, we'll move onto the digital aspect of cutting social media usage in half. That is, utilizing tools to stop using it that much. They are quite helpful for those who can't structure their days well, get rid of distractions or who aren't sure where to start. It might take you a single app (install and activate) to find the balance between using social media at the right times of the day and doing your work for the rest of the time.

Set It Up Right: Tips and Tools

Let's begin with the tips.

Turn off notifications.

You don't need these. That goes together with having intentions. As obviously, when you have the time and have decided to open a social networking site, you'll be able to spare 5-10 minutes and check what's new, but without letting that ruin your focus for the next hour or so.

Make that process easier by turning off notifications. That can be done on all channels. It might take you a few minutes to find that option in the Settings, but it's worth the time as you'll never see an alert for something that doesn't concern you anymore. Such as somebody's first story on Instagram, who of your friends on Facebook have birthdays today, an invite to a game, something recommended to you from the app itself, and so on. You don't need any of that. It will be so nice if your phone makes noises less often during the day. That will help you learn how to reach out for it only when you need it, not when you receive a notification. Because when you do, even if you just check it out, you then decide to unlock your phone and go close it, then end up on the main page of the platform, and because you're there anyway, you end up scrolling down a bit. That leads to many other actions, and gets your mind away from what you were doing.

There are a few things you can do. Let's explore the 3 areas of receiving notifications, and how to stop each.

1. Alerts from the apps themselves. - these can be turned off for any application by looking at the Settings. In the worst case, if you can't find the right button for that, search on Google 'how to turn off notifications on [add a social media site name]' and you'll see a short post, images, and videos that will help you do it in under a minute.

2. Email alerts. - for that to be removed, you can either unsubscribe from the bottom of the email the next time you receive one or visit the apps' Settings pages again and uncheck the 'Email Notifications' box.

3. Notifications from your phone. - Finally, grab your phone and say 'no' to any alert from a social media site once and for all. For an Android phone, that's as simple as going to Settings, then clicking Apps and tapping each, to see a box for notifications that you can quickly uncheck.

Note that for this action, you don't need to uninstall anything. You can still have it all on your phone, but you're limiting the power you once gave to each app, so you won't be bothered with news or updates unless you manually log in and see what's going on. Makes life easier, right?

Change your privacy.

Now, keep in mind that the founders of the biggest social media channels, as well as the investors and companies behind the smaller ones, are always looking to add new features and give you more options. But it's the paradox of choice that having more to choose from leads to more confusion and we feel worse. Life was simpler when there was one possible way to use any gadget. It's not like that anymore. Luckily, we can set it up so that our information or location isn't shared everywhere, so that we aren't given recommendations on new friends or people to follow or pages to like, and so that our profile isn't visible to people we have nothing in common with.

Let's set some boundaries by tackling the privacy settings of the social media platforms you're using daily. Assuming you already did delete an app or two and let go of it, unfollowed those you didn't want to see and turned off notifications, you can now stand up for your rights in terms of privacy.

One of the things that makes social media so powerful, is that you do what you're told, knowing everyone else is doing it and you don't want to feel left behind. So, when joining a new platform, you fill all the empty boxes given to you, and so you share where you live, where you studied, your birth date, email, and phone number, real name, and more. It wouldn't take someone more than 10 minutes to know the most important information about your life. That's just the beginning, though. If you've allowed the app to know where you are using the GPS on your phone, people can even monitor your activities. Not to mention that means never being able to tell others you won't be going out, if you just changed your plans. It's a bit scary when we're talking about our kids. Turns out, teenagers are sharing information about themselves online more often and openly as the years go by. Most have set the app to track their location automatically wherever they are and don't need to turn this off. They can easily get addicted to the feeling of connection this gives them, and so they can't go anywhere without their phone, also letting all their friends know where they are.

But most of that is what we allowed to happen, and we can take back control (partly) by making our online activities more private.

Here are some ideas on how to improve privacy and security on networking sites, and feel more comfortable sharing information with a limited number of people and knowing our behavior won't be accessible to anyone else:

Facebook

Luckily, over the past few years, Facebook gave its users more options to allow or block distractions and information flow. Although it can be a bit of a hassle if you never played with these and aren't sure what each means (and haven't decided what you want to limit exactly), it's worth taking the time to explore each item, or maybe just uncheck them all and be as private as possible.

Log in to Facebook and go to your profile. Depending on the device (desktop or mobile), and operating system you're using, these may look different. But the basics are similar.

Right now, I'm clicking the 3 dots under my profile on my Android phone. And I click 'View Privacy Shortcuts'. That takes me to the Privacy Checkup page, and from there I can choose the following:

'Who can see my stuff?' - you can make your future posts private, share them with friends or friends of friends only, or use some of the other forms of categorizations the platform is offering. I like the option to control who can see your activity log. Mine is set to 'only me'. What this means is, if I leave a comment on somebody's status, it won't immediately pop up on all my friends' timelines.

Then you'll see 'Who can contact me?' where you can choose that only friends of friends can send you friend requests.

There are more settings at the bottom of this page. After clicking that and going to the first item, 'General', you'll be able to remove your phone number from your account or turn the notifications off.

The next item on the list is 'Privacy'. This gives you some more control over your activities and information. You can decide who can look you up on Facebook using your email address (as this is something you can't delete), or using your phone number. You can also disallow search engines outside of the site to link to your profile.

Next, in 'Timeline and Tagging', you are given some more options that will help you stop feeling like every move of yours online is being watched. You can say that only friends will see the posts you're tagged in and have the chance to review anything before it appears on your timeline. You can stop random people from having the freedom to post on your wall, and so much more.

In another item below called 'Notifications', you see what we were talking about earlier and can manage it with one click. For each possible thing that you usually get notified about on Facebook, you can uncheck the 'Push' option. It's currently on. That means it won't be appearing on your phone anymore and you'll be able to breathe freely during the day when you're not actually on Facebook. From there you can also turn off all email and SMS notifications.

Now, we won't go over other platforms, but you get the point. Some people would avoid spending the next 7 minutes of their life playing with the settings when they can check updates at the same time. But it's a good investment of your time as it will save you a lot of distractions down the road, and will improve the quality of your daily life. So, do it right now. Go ahead and click the Settings of the networking site you spend the most time on daily.

Remember that nothing online is truly private. And most probably your history and all activities that you've done on each site over the years will always be accessible somehow. But unless you're a politician or have something to hide, you don't need to worry about that. The goal now is to make your future more social media-free.

Now, let me share with you the simplest and most effective software tools that will help you limit social media usage.

Tools

Before we move onto the actual list of tools, let me address your main concern about this. We're talking about disconnecting from social media and thus having a new beginning, so why would we install and use more tools to do the job? Well, that's because it's effective, and we can't argue when there are results.

There's so much we do on our smartphones every hour, that the point is to just block some of these influences for a fixed period, or until we turn them back on, so we can proceed with our day, or even take a break from networking for a few hours or even days.

The smart tools I'll now share with you, work because they do what you most probably won't do right, or easily yourself. That is, they can track your activity and give you reports, thus letting you see the big picture of what a big role social media plays in your life. You can also set limits on them, and they won't let you be tempted to log in. Some block access to sites you've checked, and you simply can't use them. Others can make social sites inaccessible by making noises, locking them, reminding you that you decided not to use these, or else. You also get notified when you exceed a daily limit. There are plenty of options, but it's important to test a few and see what works best for your needs and wants.

I'll divide the list below into 3 categories. The first items are for those wanting to track their social media usage and see what they should do next. It's good to have a more responsible online life, and that begins by seeing some numbers and time tracking. Then, the next category of tools will present you options to limit time spent on social media apps and block access. The third group will include some next level tools, for those wanting to unplug even more and see how it goes.

Most such software tools are available for both iOS and Android, but if the case is different, that will be mentioned in brackets next to each item below.

1. Monitoring Social Media Usage.

BreakFree - tracks how long you stay on your phone and suggests when it's time to take a break.

QualityTime (for Android) - this one works in the background, tracking the amount of time during which the phone is unlocked, and which apps are used the most. You can set it to give you alerts if you exceed the time. It reports some interesting numbers, such as how many times you unlocked the phone, how many minutes you spent on each platform, what time of the day you're most active, or even how many times you logged in to an app. These numbers can be scary if we never thought about it. What I love the most about QualityTime, though, is that you can click 'Take a Break' and your phone will freeze for a set amount of time. Great for doing some uninterrupted work and not being tempted to check your phone.

Moment (for iOS) - install the app on your iPhone, set it up and forget about it. It will help you use your phone less. See which apps you use the most, and set daily limits to receive notifications such as reminders.

StayOnTask (for Android) - this one won't be pushy at all, and will just gently ask you if you're focused on your work, to remind you not to get distracted with your phone or other things. It has some simple but effective features such as scheduling times to start tracking work sessions automatically, changing alarm tones, and adjusting the frequency of reminders during work, and during the rest of the time.

2. Blocking Apps.

Offtime - get access only to the things you need (by choosing some of the modes it offers), and forget about anything else such as games and social media. It has smart app blocking, communication filters, and reports on how you're spending your time on your phone.

AppDetox (for Android) - this one is for taking a digital detox by setting some parameters for each app, and having access to them only when you're not busy with something more important.

FocusON (for Android) - this tool can block anything you think is a distraction, either for a certain amount of time or schedule it for different days.

ClearLock (for Android) - simply block all apps on your device that you wish to spend less time on, and set some limits as to how long that should continue.

ColdTurkey - this smart tool first tells you what you're using the most on your phone, and then asks you what you'd like to have less access to and for how long. If you try to enter one of the blocked apps during that period, you'll see the site is unavailable.

3. A more aggressive approach to blocking.

Flipd (for Android) - feeling annoyed by the fact that you're using a social site too much, and want to do something right away to remove the distraction? Well, this app takes it to the next level by letting you lock your phone for a certain amount of time. Then there's nothing you can do about it until that moment comes and you gain access again, not even restarting your phone will help.

StepLock - want to ditch social media and get active instead? Here's an app that makes you do it. StepLock makes you exercise to use your favorite apps again. It's an innovative self-control tool. You set the numbers in the beginning, and then it will track your steps. When the goal is reached, the apps are unblocked again.

Forest - turns ditching social media into a game. You receive rewards, can track things and measure progress, compete with friends and stay motivated. You're basically growing a tree when you open and activate it, and thus take responsibility by staying there and not opening social media sites. It's an interesting approach and includes mindfulness and a sense of achievement.

Now you have all the strategies, methods and tools of a mindful social media user in your hands. Time to put them into practice.

Disconnect, But Keep in Touch

Before moving onto the chapter on how to completely disconnect and get rid of social media once and for all, thus welcoming a new life with a clear mind and better communication, let's discuss the last bits about partial unplugging. That is - after seeing how to set limits to your social media usage, change your habits, embrace mindfulness before, during and after being online, and using the help of some smart tools - you should also know how to keep in touch with friends, even if you're there for them less often or for shorter periods of time.

How Not to Get Anyone Offended

There's the possibility of affecting your relationship with your friends in a negative way if you don't take precautions. Your social media decluttering isn't what most people would decide to do, even at a later stage in their life, so keep in mind they won't necessarily understand your reasons.

If they don't know your 'why', they can easily assume you're looking for ways to avoid communicating with them. They might think you're being cold, or don't seem to care about them as much as you did before. When, in reality, you're just changing your habits as a social media user and clearing your mind.

Well, the simplest way to avoid any misunderstanding is to explain your reasons clearly. So, get on the social media channel where you keep in contact with your most important people. Take some time to write a longer message, sharing your plan with them and giving details such as when you'll be available and how it's best to connect you from here on. Let them know this is important to you and part of your personal development journey and your new beginning as a more productive, focused and successful individual. Also, do tell your friends in this message that their support would mean a lot and they will help you make this change more easily if they don't take it personally.

Usually, that's enough to get them to contact you less often, or just be okay with you responding when you decide it's time for that and after you've done your most important work for the day.

Make Your Time on Social Media Count

What about when you log in and it's time to answer all messages, check some notifications, grab some inspiration from here and there, or leave a comment? Well, do this with a purpose and enjoy it.

73

The keyword phrase here should be 'meaningful communication'. That's your main point for using your phone anyways. Anything else might easily trick you back into old patterns and you'll get distracted and upset again.

Here are some tips on how to do that:

> Log in and go directly into the messaging area, or type the name of the friend you want to contact and say what you have to;

> If the person isn't online, don't wait. Just write what's on your mind and leave. Otherwise, you'll kill the time till they check their phone by reading stuff that shouldn't be part of your day;

> Never scroll down a feed if you still haven't limited what's on it;

> Ideally, use just an app like Messenger (not Facebook itself), WhatsApp or Viber. There you have only the contact details of people you communicate with often, and can choose not to read anything from those who aren't part of your current life. Such apps give enough privacy to talk about personal stuff and know nothing will be public;

> Ditch messaging and call a friend once a day. That's real-time communication. Texting prevents you from being an active listener, and you end up missing important details and not making your conversations count;

> To keep a relationship going do video calls once or twice a week. Seeing each other changes everything. Even if you

don't have anything new to share, just talk about what you're currently doing and how your day is going.

Create rituals with your best friends, relatives in other countries, or partner who's away every now and then. For instance, know when both of you are available and have a fixed hour every third or so day, to have a 15-minute call. Could be multitasking as well, if you're walking, the other person is on the treadmill or commuting. Make sure you stick to this for the first few calls, and then it will be your new thing. You two will feel guilty if you can't make it to the call and might leave something else you have to do for later, to make an appearance on the social media channel. Such a ritual might sound stupid when you explain the whole idea to a friend who's just doing things on the spur of the moment. But it can make or break a relationship over time. Just give this a try, and you'll enjoy the communication online and will be looking forward to the next call. What's more, you won't be contacting each other for every little thing during the day and often bothering each other during work hours, or in unexpected stressful situations. But will just share it all when the time for a call comes. That also brings balance;

Use social media to arrange real meetings. It's a free tool to connect with people wherever you are, and whenever you feel like. So, utilize it by suggesting an hour and date for a meeting that works for you, and see their reaction. If they can't, after a few more lines you'll come to an agreement and will meet soon. But be the initiator as it's easy to just start chatting about random things and avoid going out and spending some face-to-face time.

That's how you can disconnect and keep in touch. Pretty straightforward, right?

Now, all that we discussed in chapter 2 can transform your life pretty soon. If you start with ditching one bad phone habit, trying one new method for mindful social media usage, and setting one limitation as to how, when and how much you use it, you'll feel like a new you in a week.

The first 3 days will be hard. It will feel awkward. You'll crave social media like you crave sugar when you're on a strict diet. But these signals are fake. It's the symptoms of addiction showing, and your mind wants what it's used to. But it's best for it if you restrain. Just do it for a day. Tell yourself that each morning, and feel good about following through in the evening. It gets easier with each next day. A detailed plan will be your best friend in moments of despair.

Part 3

Disconnect Completely

If you made it to the third and final chapter, congrats. You now completely understand how dangerous social media can be and that it's time for a new beginning.

Maybe you already gave the mindful social media usage approach a try. And maybe it was successful, and you liked the feeling of control over your free time and the peace of mind that you got in return. Now you most probably want more of it, and so you're here waiting to see the step-by-step plan below that will help you get rid of this once and for all.

It's time to disconnect.

Why would someone do that if they don't have a serious problem with being stuck to their phones 24/7? Here are a few reasons.

Quitting it makes you happier.

If you leave social media for good, you'll boost your happiness and get your life back. Multiple studies have shown the effect abandoning it has on your mind and soul, but also your anxiety issues, signs of depression and low self-esteem. Quite many people share things like:

> Ditching social media helped them feel less like a failure;

> It made them enjoy their day-to-day life more (as you don't feel the pressure of having to upload a picture when you're at a restaurant, for instance, and then await responses. Instead, your phone won't play a key role in your day anymore and you'll just do things and enjoy them.);

> Many young people say platforms like Facebook don't tempt them anymore as literally everyone's there and it feels crowded. So, they take a break from it, are surprised by how much they don't need to log back in, and just never do it;

> Individuals also share that life without social media as a big factor makes them more positive. They don't worry about what others think anymore and that liberates them, giving them the freedom to engage their mind in better things;

> You forget about the fake needs that arise when you're a frequent social media user. These are things such as the need for attention, having to share your life online, to stay updated, to answer to everybody and check notifications, to be prompted to give more information on your profile or join new platforms, to know a ton of stuff about random people just because they're always online, to be frustrated as to what the norm is and to try and follow trends, to be judged and to judge without realizing it, to have to prove yourself, etc.

It's not as hard to quit it as you might think.

If you tell somebody who's been using social media for years to just leave it, delete accounts, stop answering to people, and never check their phone too many times in a day again, they'll think you're crazy for even proposing that. They think they can't just stop using it, without having thought about it, without a plan, etc. What's more, their mind immediately comes up with tens of reasons as to how much they need it, love it and why it's a good thing. Be it for social or personal reasons. Of course, that's the illusion they live with and the virtual world. The 24/7 connection, the fear of missing out, the desire to fit in, are all contributing to the fake reality they've created for themselves.

However, quitting doesn't need to be hard. It's about understanding the main principles behind using social media (which were already laid out earlier in the book), and that we do it for the wrong reasons. It's about seeing its bad effect on all areas of our life, and how good and free it could be without it.

After that, it will be like breaking any bad old habit. With a plan in mind, and reminding yourself of why you're better off without the behavior, you can quit it in no time and never look back.

Most people who did it are amazed at how easier life is when they don't need to check for updates every 30 minutes. When their free time is literally free.

You start doing better things with your time.

The only way to find out what else you could be doing with your time and what productivity really means, is to disappear from social media and just forget about it.

For a start, you'll begin thinking about better things other than what you saw on your feed or who you're chatting about random stuff with. Then, you will be more mindful of your present moment will now be free and you can pay your attention to it, thus enjoying life a bit more.

Some time after not being a social media user, you'll notice some nice changes. Such as that you're generating more ideas, are keeping yourself busy and always doing something, thus feeling more accomplished at the end of the day. You won't be late anymore because of staring at your phone and losing track of time. And when you walk or do something else, you'll be focused on the activity instead of multitasking with your phone in your hand.Such a new approach to doing everything will show results at school, work and with your personal goals. Expect to see more progress than ever, with whatever it is that you're doing.

The other forms of communication feel way better.

There's no chance to see what true communication is and how it feels like to connect with somebody if you still rely on social media.

I'm talking about the chance of getting to know a new student or colleague face to face during lunch break. That wouldn't happen if you're both staring at your phones, or just add each other on Facebook and never really connect.

Or how about learning big news about friends and relatives when meeting somewhere? That's a much more genuine way to be happy about them and be pleasantly surprised. When that's on social media, it's usually in the form of a status they post, which we see in a time of the day when we can't really call them. Later we can either message them to say 'Congrats!' or something like that, or just forget about it as a lot more has happened since then.

Now, before we get to the plan I've promised you on how to get out of social media, and never need to come back again, let me share how I did it exactly.

How I Completely Disconnected Myself from Social Media, and Why It Was Great

I remember the day I took the final decision to do it. I had just wasted another morning on my phone, without having a chance to get ready for the day, have some quiet time or get out on time. All that, even though I was waking up earlier than I had to.

Also, I caught myself doing some of the following things during the day:

> Not being interested in a conversation with the person in front of me, but dying to check my phone and chat;

> Needing 10 minutes to get back to work after I've logged in on any of the channels I was using. I did that often, so imagine the ridiculously small amount of time I spent being focused on work;

> I was feeling anxious when I hadn't checked Facebook for a few hours. When I finally get to it, there's a moment of satisfaction, followed by boredom;

I sometimes spent a minute here or there reading comments under a post which didn't concern me at all. I always realized that but did it anyway, which also made me feel out of control of my mind and action. That didn't contribute to my confidence.

All these often made me frustrated, angry for being weak, overwhelmed with a ton of emotions all of which seemed so insignificant compared to the real things in life.

I started journaling and that helped a lot. I wanted to internalize the reasons why I did all that, and even though there's a deeper reason for everything, here the solution seemed obvious. I knew that if I managed to get out of social media once and for all, my life would take a better direction.

Then, I decided to read one story about a person who did it successfully every morning for a few days. On my laptop, not phone. It's great to see how many of them shared it on their personal blogs or even made it to big publications. I'm talking about famous internet personalities, or just average people, some with their own businesses too, who saw the effect of social media on their minds and lives and said the big 'no'. Some did it for a month just to see how it goes and loved the results. Others never logged in again on any of the channels that were once their favorite. But none of them complained about it.

I needed this motivation boost as a reminder. To see it's possible to do it, even if you're working online, have many friends you want to keep in touch with, or have been a big fan of social media since you can remember. In all these cases, people determined to see life without this negative behavior were happy with the outcome.

What you do first thing in the morning is crucial. And so, because I was feeding my mind with motivation like that, it was a matter of time till I was ready to commit the social media suicide. Now, some try and prepare for too long, during which time they are still being available on all channels. That wasn't how I wanted to do it.

I did first try all the things I described in the previous chapter and thus became a mindful social media user. But because I loved it so much and wanted to challenge myself by taking this experiment to the next level, I made a plan on how to do the ultimate social media escape.

Stop preparing, just do it.

Usually, that's the easiest way. Slow progress and preparation are great for other things, but here you need to go through the first few days as quickly as possible so that you can start seeing the benefits I mentioned at the beginning of the book.

What to expect in the first few days.

Simply said, there will be withdrawal symptoms. If you're doing it after trying most of the mindfulness techniques covered in the previous chapter, then it will be easier. But be ready to notice all awkward signs of addiction and to be willing to resist the urges.

In my case, it looked like this:

I'd unlock my phone and be on the verge of opening Facebook or Instagram before I realize I deleted them and I'm actually in the process of breaking the social media habit.

I would often stop what I'm doing for a moment, and think about what's missing. Then, remember it's the lack of phone alerts about new notifications or messages. I'd laugh about this and get back to my things. Every time that happened, I was grateful I'm making this change and breaking free from the trap I was in.

I was often bored but knew well it was just the lack of comfort that the constant stream of information gave me. So now that I was back to reality, I had to entertain myself in other ways.

It works to read stuff on your computer. There's still news to be heard, interesting blogs to read, or even people to follow. But it doesn't need to be on social media or by using your phone.

Then, people started noticing. Some called to ask why I haven't been online for more than 12 hours on Facebook, others wanted to know if I had changed my number on WhatsApp. I had a lot of explaining to do and had to stay patient.

Later came the moment when colleagues started asking me about stuff going on social media, that I had obviously missed. I was okay with that but was a bit anxious and wanted them to stop talking about it.

The hard part is that you can eliminate the temptation itself by deleting your accounts. But you can't stop others from using it, so you see it everywhere.

Then, you start doing other things.

I kept journaling how I felt every day, what I missed, and reminding myself (by writing again) that it was the right thing to do and I'm going to be enjoying a better life soon. And that's exactly what happened.

I started reading books when commuting. I began talking to people more, at home, at work and just everywhere outside. Communication was easier now. Before that, it was a bit of an effort and social media just seemed like the simpler solution.

I also felt like calling friends and asking them out. Every time it led to a better connection than ever before. They supported me in my decision to stop using social media and some even saw improvement in me and were a bit jealous of me having one less thing to think about.

I finally organized my days better. Had my to-do list written down the night before or first thing in the morning. Set some goals and wrote them down. Kept my email inbox empty. These are little things but contributed to my productivity throughout the whole day.

It became easier for me to get to work right away, regardless of what I was doing before that. One huge distraction was removed, and I was enjoying the increased energy and focus.

In the beginning, I felt a bit guilty for having deleted all my accounts. The need to check them was obvious. I felt like installing the apps again many times. But then it suddenly became better without them. I wasn't sure why in the first days, but after a week I was able to write it all out in my journal and feel good about what I had done.

I want you to experience the same. It's amazing how disconnection leads to connection. And doing less leads to doing more.

I'll now share with you what exact actions to take to detach from social media.

Your Step-by-Step Plan on Cutting Social Media for Good

Let me begin by this: you're not alone. Enough people have realized (and are doing it at this very moment) how social media usage ruins our health, peace of mind and ability to live normally and succeed. In fact, a survey shows that in 2017 more people are looking to break this bad habit rather than to quit smoking.

You can take each of the following steps in the order given, and once a day for the next 5 days.

1. Set 30 minutes aside to think it through.

Every new beginning starts with some thinking, brainstorming, and planning. And although all that you already read the book so far let you come to some important conclusions and see things from another perspective, you still have some things to decide. Such as:

- Who do you need to tell before you quit social media? - Make sure the people you communicate with regularly are aware of this and let them know how you'll keep in touch from here on.

- Fix possible issues regarding work. - There might be a group you joined, or a page that informs you about what's going on at work, school, or with something important you care about. Find other ways to receive the key information without having to be on social media for it.

- Write down some phone numbers, or other info that might come in handy soon, but which you checked only on social media so far. Could be birthdays of friends, dates that matter for your company or family, or else.

- Think of possible issues that can arise from your absence on social media. Will someone get offended? Have you promised to do something that can only happen on social media?

2. Delete all your accounts aside from the ones you use the most.

You might want to keep your profile on LinkedIn for networking purposes and career opportunities. It's not really a place for distractions either. But say goodbye to Twitter, Instagram, Snapchat, Pinterest, Tumblr, and Google Plus.

You might even want to give it a few days once you delete these (not just uninstall but remove your profiles from such platforms), and take the journey to leaving social media a bit slower.

3. Get rid of everything but 1 or 2 messaging apps.

Yes, that means you can still have Messenger, but not Facebook. Luckily, that's possible too. There's a 'Not on Facebook?' option once Messenger is installed, and you can simply use your name and phone number. That lets you stay away from the clutter but be able to chat with Facebook friends at the same time. But even if you choose to do that, you must have unfollowed all annoying pages with too much information that doesn't concern you, must have stopped notifications and deleted friends who aren't somebody you'd chat with, etc.

Now, it's up to you whether you'll leave one or two messaging apps on your phone or remove that too in a day or a few. The best way to take a decision is to see how you feel about it once you're left just with these. If you can easily do without them, remove these too. But in most cases, people can text or call only the important figures in their life, and let this be a way to save money too by relying on the Internet connection.

4. Replace using social media with something else.

You need to do something when the urge to log in again comes. That same time probably won't be spent just doing anything, as this way you'll be thinking about social media and might start using up your willpower soon.

The first few days of the disconnection are crucial for how things will go from here on. So, no chance to skip a day, as that will lead to a second one and a third one. You take a final decision to quit this habit, and never look back again.

So, what else can you be doing the next few days after you're left with just a messaging app and have no feeds to scroll or notifications to check?

Here are some ideas:

- **Read.** - Seriously, go back to reading. Could be books, blogs, or anything else that makes you feel good, engages your brain, leads to generating ideas and learning stuff.

- **Get your life in order.** - Get rid of things at home you don't use. You'll feel freer and will have more space for new and better things, not just in your house but also in your mind. Then, organize everything and have a place for each item at home. Use lists for all that needs to be done so you won't need to remember anymore. Add important things to your calendar. Clean your room often and keep it tidy. Never leave dirty dishes in the sink. Keep your email inbox empty too, either by answering it all in the morning, or doing it 2 or 3 times a day. Fix what's broken at home, or replace it with something new. All this won't happen in a day, of course, but it's a nice project for your 'me time' when your phone won't be of much help without apps on it.

- **Take a daily walk.** - That's great for your mental health and is a natural way to reduce stress, boost your mood and stay active.

- **Start meditating.** - All you need is an isolated place and a few minutes of silence. There's nothing complicated to meditation, but it's a sure way to find peace in life and be able to handle problems more easily. It's beneficial to your health too, keeps you alert and mentally and emotionally healthy.

- **Start a blog and publish your first blog post.** - Writing is fun if you give it a go. Many people are scared to share their thoughts with the world, but it can start small and lead to something big. If you have stuff in your mind that you want to get out, begin blogging and experience its benefits.

- **Call a friend.** - You might feel uncomfortable doing that if you are used to just chatting with people, but this will feel great and you won't regret it.

- **Do things you've been putting off for a long time.** - Such list is usually somewhere in the back of our minds, and we avoid getting to it and indulge in things such as social media instead. Now, however, you can face all that you've said 'no' to but which must be done.

- **Prep a meal.** - Get even more organized by preparing your meals when you have the time for it so that you won't need to grab junk food later in the day.

- **Visit more meaningful websites.** - There's a lot on the Internet that can help you in different ways. Check Udemy for online courses on something you always found interesting. Read famous people's biographies online and get inspired. Watch YouTube videos on how to do stuff in daily life that you find difficult. Read smart answers to all kinds of questions on sites like Quora. Watch TED talks to hear what some of the most brilliant people on the planet have to say and change your perspective.

These are things you can start with when you find yourself not knowing what to do with your 10 or 30 minutes of free time here and there during the day. Once you do give these different activities a try, you'll come up with many more ideas on what else to do. Eventually, you'll be making the most of every minute, will be productive instead of just keeping yourself busy, will expand your mind and will have fun at the same time.

5. Start a new hobby.

Taking this transformation to the next level. Time to start a new hobby to not just break a bad habit and have more time, but also build a successful new one and make the most of it.

That could be working out. Even if you're a gym goer already, you now have the focus to take sport more seriously. That means researching and understanding more about how the body builds muscles, making changes to your workout routine, adding new exercises, moving cardio from before the weight lifting part to the end, deciding to eat something in particular before or after a workout, learning about natural supplements, adding more proteins and veggies to your diet to make the most of your gym session for the day, checking out new gym gear, etc.

You also have the chance to go back to an old hobby and be more invested in it this time. Think about something you always enjoyed, which came naturally to you, and which made you lose track of time. Might be cooking, taking pictures, writing, or else. Make it part of your days again.

If you're up for something new that will also help you see progress in other areas of life, then think of learning a new language and getting familiar with a new culture. Or take an online course to learn a skill that can be monetized, such as programming, web design or affiliate marketing.

By doing one such thing, together with the little things that will replace social media usage during the day, you can become more productive, creative, successful and driven. That will lead to beautiful changes in your life and will shape your future.

That's how the steps of quitting social media forever really look like. Together with all the tips you saw in the previous chapters, you now have the knowledge and plan to act today.

Tips on How to Stay Consistent

When you start a new behavior without enough preparation or a plan on how to do it long enough without any obstacles and simply give up, you soon realize that it's hard to keep going. But without being consistent in this, you won't see results. The quick benefits you can notice by taking a break from social media can easily disappear if you go back to your normal routine shortly after. That's why we'll now discuss what comes after building a new habit - the part where you make it a permanent element of your life.

Here are some tips. It's worth reading them right before day 1 of your social media escape (when you'll put the plan you read above into action). Following the advice below will also make your journey easier as you'll be prepared for the moments when things might go wrong.

1. Give your plan a deadline.

Our mind works much better when we give it an end date for a new venture. That's for a few reasons.

To begin with, we work well under pressure. A <u>deadline serves as a motivator</u> to get the work done before the due date, and makes us think more creatively too. That's why entrepreneurs know they should give assignments with deadlines to their workers. Because this makes them work more effectively, keeps them focused and distractions are less likely to occur now that there's a goal to be achieved in a certain time period.

Second, a deadline in our case can be a milestone. We're making a lifelong change here, and we want permanent results. So, we'll set deadlines for each phase of this project. That would be the social media break first, followed by the beginning of the ultimate disconnection, one step at a time, according to the plan provided.

Such milestones keep it interesting as we are challenged. Time pressure, in such situations, doesn't allow us to lead astray and just leave things behind for a day or two. Then we'll feel like a failure.

And that's when yet another benefit of this simple technique comes - completing each small deadline feels like a win. That gives us proof that we can keep going and see even bigger progress, and gives us the satisfaction that we need to find joy in the process and feel good about ourselves.

Deadlines are powerful. But with lifestyle changes, you're the one who needs to set them for yourself. Do some brainstorming now and write down some dates and numbers. Keep it realistic as you don't want to overwhelm yourself.

With the goal of stopping social media usage, deadlines may look like this:

- Write down your plan for a life without social media, and delete accounts you're not using that much in the next 4 days;

- For the next week, wake up and immediately start doing something else, so that you don't check your phone in the first hour of the morning;

- Practice social media mindfulness by using only one or more messaging apps, only when you need it, and put your phone away right after you've said what you had to, instead of waiting for a response and checking feeds during that time;

- In the next 2 days, send a well-thought-out message to each friend you keep in touch with, explaining what you're going to do and how you can be reached when necessary.

These are some examples that work well. Of course, don't set more than 1 deadline at a time, as it can feel unpleasant to limit yourself that much. Which brings me to the next point on the list...

2. One change at a time.

We're trying to do something big here. To set ourselves free from one of our worst habits and one of the most negative influences in modern life. So that won't happen as quickly as we'd like it to. I'll ask you to be patient. And in order not to wait for fast results, then get disappointed and ditch the whole plan, you'll need to make your steps and actions as small as you can.

Remember this: take one small step at a time.

That means you can't follow all the tips above, as each requires some other changes, breaking old habits or starting new behaviors, coming to some realizations and restricting yourself a bit. If you go for it all, your willpower will end soon, and you'll be left with a void inside, that only social media might fill. Let's not get to that dark place, and instead stay consistent with this.

3. Give yourself 21 days.

Experts say it takes 21 days to adjust to a new behavior and consider the new habit formed. After that, it's easier to keep doing this, although temptations will be everywhere around as you can't stop others from being attached to their phones too.

So, let this be your first big deadline, among the small ones you'll have in-between. 3 weeks is a great time period to track. Simply getting a calendar and putting an X for each day you spend without wasting time on networking sites, is a step closer to your big goal.

It's scientifically proven that after the initial 21 days, your brain has been exposed to the new lifestyle enough, to make it easier for you to continue this way without investing too much willpower anymore. You should be cautious again, of course, for weeks and even months after you've given up social media. But it will be much easier to deal with the urges.

4. Get someone else on board with you.

There's little to no chance a good friend of yours will be making this same lifestyle change at the same time. But you can propose it to somebody who's looking to improve their mental health, wants a challenge, or is looking for a way to simplify their life and reduce stress.

For them, the experiment might just be 2 weeks or a month, but that will still be beneficial to their lives, and you'll get the support you need for the first stage of your battle.

If you can't find anyone to do that with you, then seek such people in online communities. There are enough forums, blogs, and groups out there for people trying to achieve any goal you can think of. And they motivate each other to stay strong in the face of doubt and distraction.

5. Don't be a perfectionist.

Perfectionism can kill your dreams. The desire to change, improve and even thrive with something hard such as removing social media from your life, will be impossible to keep if you want everything to be perfect. No. You'll have your weak moments and might even fail to completely stop using social sites a few times. But then you need to try again and have more information about what might go wrong this time.

Also, you might end up indulging in another behavior you wouldn't like, such as eating a bit more, thinking about social media and looking at others using it, getting a bit depressed because of the illusion of connection it's been giving you, and more.

These struggles will go away, just give it time. And be okay with mistakes and imperfections.

6. Look at it as an experiment.

There's a cool mind trick you can try in order not to feel overwhelmed by the big picture. After all, it might sound scary to think about deleting many accounts, having more free time on your hands, having to use your phone less, not having anything better to do while walking or during lunch break, etc. So, don't think about all this. Instead, do this as an experiment, or a challenge.

It's about getting out of your comfort zone, using more of your potential now that social media won't be affecting your thinking, and doing better things with your time.

Shift your mindset and start thinking that you're getting better and better at this with every next day, that you finally have the focus you needed to excel at your job, start training more seriously or monetize your hobby.

7. Know the bad side of what you're doing.

I helped you imagine all the benefits you'll experience by not having social media dictate your life anymore earlier in the book. But I also presented to you some negative scenarios, such as how addicted to it we might get, how hard it was for me to ditch it and the emptiness I was feeling, and the possibility of failing as we are too used to it. That's realistic and it's better if you know this.

Getting yourself familiar with what might go wrong, or what others have experienced as side effects, is useful information that will help you recognize the patterns when or if they occur.

Meaning, you might feel a bit isolated a few days after you delete a social media account that you've been using for years now. But by knowing this is supposed to happen, you'll remind yourself it's normal and it's a fake feeling caused by the kind of socializing you were doing on these networks.

By doing that, you'll find it easier to let go and do something else with your time instead, thus focusing your mind on more productive activities.

8. Breathe and be free.

Finally, I want to remind you to enjoy the process of what you're doing, even before you've seen the actual advantages in real life, and before others around you notice the wonderful transformation you're going through.

No social media allows you to live more fully. But to do that, you should practice mindfulness, while away from any device. That means stopping a few times throughout the day, taking a few deep breaths, and just spending some time in the moment, noticing how great everything you have and do is, and not having to change anything about it.

Do that daily, and you'll become a happier person. Such happiness is contagious.

Conclusion

If you made it to the end of the book, congrats and thank you for starting this journey. You're making the world a better place by being a role model, living a more mindful and productive life, making the right decisions, and not preferring technology over reality.

I can't wait for you to see how this new beginning looks like exactly. There's no better way than to try it for yourself, starting today.

Take that social media break for a few days, see how it goes, analyze the results and plan how to make it easier for yourself when following the actual plan for disconnection.

I began this book by talking about our attention and how multiple factors try to take it away from us, thus making us live a life we don't really feel satisfied with. Social media is one of these influences, and by removing it you're getting your attention back.

Once you have control over it, you can change your direction, and finally, do all that you've ever dreamed of. Working on a new project that might shape your future is one way to use this extra time and focus. But you can also just dedicate these to forming real connections with loved ones, spending more time in their company, and smiling during any activity in the day, no matter how simple it is, because now you can genuinely enjoy it, when there's no phone in your hand and unnecessary thoughts in your mind anymore.

New beginnings are exciting. We can't even predict all the positive things that will happen as a result of one such change. And that's why this guide will help you tremendously. It shares part of my journey to breaking this bad habit, but also gives room for personalization. You'll tailor this towards your needs, will do it your way, for your own reasons, and will enjoy the benefits in different ways. And that's alright.

You'll soon get your attention back. That makes you more powerful than half of the population in the world. Think carefully what you're going to do with these powers and how you can use them to your advantage. Do more meaningful things with your time. But don't forget to enjoy the small ups and downs of life during the day, as it's what makes us who we are.

This new beginning doesn't need to be your last one either. It's the ultimate beginning, to all other beginnings. Transformations happen in phases, and that's your starting line. Once you make a change such as to stop using social media, it gets easier with anything else down the road.

The principles of change remain the same, regardless of what it is you're trying to achieve. Removing one bad behavior and replacing it with a good one, teaches you lessons like no degree or person can. You experience it for yourself, get to know how your mind and body work, take control over your actions, develop the mindset of a winner, and can only move forward from there on.

Life is about new beginnings. But we aren't aware of that until we have one. Each is life-changing, making us better people, liberating us from negative factors, and letting us enter a reality of higher quality, one that we created for ourselves and which is exactly how we like it.

Over to you know. Time to put all that you read about into practice.

What's different about you since you opened that book and now that you've gone through it? What's your first step? What important realizations did you come to while reading? Did you highlight parts which you'll come back to or did you take notes already? Do you have a plan in mind on how to stop social media for good? And are you excited about your new life without it?

You can help me and your fellow readers by leaving a review on Amazon and sharing your thoughts on this book. You have no idea how much this would help!

One last thing. How would you like winning **a $200.00 Amazon Gift Card** and helping me improve this book in the process with a little bit of feedback?

That's right :)

Your opinion is so valuable to me that I am giving away a $200 gift card to the *luckiest one of 200 participants*!

It will only take a minute of your time to let me know what you like and what you didn't like about this book. The hardest part is deciding how to spend the two hundred dollars!

Just follow this link.

http://booksfor.review/quittingsocial

About the Author:

Lidiya K is an author and blogger in the fields of personal, spiritual and business growth. She's the creator of Let's Reach Success and self-publishes eBooks all the time.

She's all about lifestyle design and aspires to make a statement with her words, actions and business.

[this page is intentionally left blank]

26126851R00066

Printed in Great Britain
by Amazon